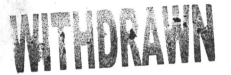
Help! Does my patient know more than me?

Report of a conference held jointly by the King's Fund and the
Enabling People Programme
16 March 1999

Nancy Kohner
Alison Hill

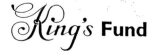
King's Fund

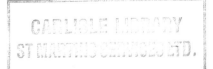

Published by
King's Fund Publishing
11–13 Cavendish Square
London W1M 0AN

ISBN 1 85717 401 1

A CIP catalogue record for this book is available from the British Library

Available from:

King's Fund Bookshop
11–13 Cavendish Square
London
W1M 0AN

Tel: 020 7307 2591
Fax: 020 7307 2801

Printed and bound in Great Britain

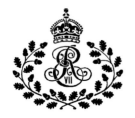

Contents

Foreword

Julia Neuberger, Chief Executive, King's Fund

The political climate in which information is made available to patients is changing. We now have a patient population which is much better informed – not necessarily, or only, by health professionals but also through the media and the Internet. This information may not always be good quality, but there can be no uncertainty about the quantity that is available.

The quality of information is a complicating factor. Patients will not necessarily be able to understand the information they have access to, nor distinguish what is relevant, useful and reliable.

A further complication is the age differential. Younger service users are, on the whole, likely to be better informed than older ones, not only because they have the skills to access information but also because of changing attitudes towards the role of the health care professional. While some older people may still believe that health professionals should fulfil a paternalistic role, younger people increasingly see health professionals as advisers offering expert advice which they, as service users, may or may not choose to follow. This changing relationship between user and professional directly affects what information is given and the way it is communicated.

The title of this conference, 'Help! Does my patient know more than me?' reflects the professional insecurity created by these changes. But patient information is not just the concern of individual professionals. Although we understand much more now than we ever did about making information accessible to people at an individual level, we do not yet understand very much about why, in our organisation or practice, we may sometimes, apparently deliberately, make information obscure or hard to get at.

This conference, and the study of which it is a part, address both these issues: the way in which information is handled at the individual level, within the consultation, for example; and the way in which organisations need to change in order to make information available and accessible to users.

Introduction

In 1998, a multi-centre study was set up to identify the learning needs of clinicians and the organisational changes required if patients' information needs are to be fulfilled. The study was funded by the Enabling People Programme and involved the Universities of Glasgow, Birmingham and Nottingham, Great Ormond Street Hospital, and the King's Fund. This report describes a conference held jointly by the King's Fund and the Enabling People Programme towards the end of the programme of study.

Prior to the conference, three stages of the study had been completed:

- Interviews had been carried out with twenty clinicians in Glasgow. The taped interviews were analysed to identify learning needs and organisational changes that would help in meeting patients' information needs, mostly as perceived by clinicians.

- A revised interview was used with fifty-two clinicians in Nottingham and London.

- Using the Delphi technique and a postal questionnaire, consensus was sought among a further thirty-seven clinicians concerning the relative importance of the identified aims. Work was also started on the development of seminars and discussion groups for students and a model for self-identification of learning needs.

The conference was designed as part of the development and dissemination phase of the study and provided an opportunity to present the findings of, and issues raised by, the study to an invited, multi-professional audience, along with presentations offering complementary information and perspectives. Conference delegates were drawn from a wide range of disciplines and included researchers, educationalists, informaticists and health professionals. The conference provided a forum for debate and a means of obtaining opinion on the research findings from a mixed and experienced audience.

Conference programme

9.30 – 9.40	**Welcome and introduction**
	Julia Neuberger, Chief Executive, King's Fund

9.40 – 10.00	**Setting the scene – first principles**
	Scene-setting drama

10.00 – 10.45	**First session: What are the key issues?**
	Chair: Mrs Jean Mossman, Chief Executive, CancerBACUP
	Speakers: Dr Angela Coulter, Director, Policy and Development, King's Fund
	Ms Sally Tweddle, Senior CRC Fellow in Cancer Information and Education, University of Birmingham
	Dr Mandy Hampshire, Lecturer in General Practice, University of Nottingham and General Practitioner

10.45 – 11.00	**Coffee**

11.00 – 12.15	**Syndicate groups**

12.15 – 1.00	**Feedback**

1.00 – 2.00	**Lunch**

2.00 – 2.30	**Second session: Putting the learning into action**
	Chair: Dr David Percy, Director, Education and Training, NHS Executive, South East Regional Office
	Speakers: Dr Fiona Moss, Associate Dean, Postgraduate Medicine, North Thames
	Dr Ray Jones, Senior Lecturer in Health Informatics, University of Glasgow

2.30 – 3.30   **Syndicate groups and tea**

3.30 – 4.00   **Feedback**

4.00 – 4.15   **Summary of the day**
                    Professor Marshall Marinker, Visiting Professor of General
                    Practice, The Guy's, King's College and St Thomas Hospitals
                    Medical and Dental School, London

What are the key issues?

Patients as partners in clinical decision-making: the wider context

Summary of a presentation by Dr Angela Coulter, Director, Policy and Development, King's Fund.

There is a wealth of evidence to show that lack of information and poor communication are prime causes of patients' complaints, that doctors frequently underestimate patients' information needs, and that a large and increasing number of patients want to be actively involved in decision-making about their care. While some patients do not seek this kind of involvement, they still want their ideas, values and preferences to be taken into account in decisions that are made, although professionals may not be skilled in eliciting these.[1]

There is also some evidence that patient involvement improves the effectiveness of clinical care.[2]

Patients want information:

- about what is wrong, with clear explanations
- about the processes and likely outcomes of tests and treatments
- which will give them a realistic idea of their prognosis
- about available services, including options and alternatives
- which will reassure them
- to help others around them (family, friends, carers) to understand
- to help them identify other sources of information.[1]

Wennberg's studies of the variations in the uptake of common surgical operations revealed that the views, values and preferences of health professionals are a key determinant.[3] This finding highlights the need to build the patient's values and preferences into the decision-making process. In order to learn what the patient wants and make the correct treatment choice for the individual, the patient must be asked to participate in a process that disentangles what the patient wants from what the doctor or other caregiver may want.

Models for the decision-making process are:

- the paternalistic model, in which the clinician makes a decision on the patient's behalf
- the professional-as-agent model, in which the clinician elicits the patient's views and makes a decision which takes these views into account
- the model of shared decision-making, in which information is shared and a decision made jointly
- the model of informed decision-making (the patient choice model), in which the clinician supplies information and the patient makes the decision.

The appropriate decision-making process will vary according to the situation.

Shared decision-making is often appropriate because it offers the possibility of shared responsibility. It involves at least two (and maybe more) participants, the patient and the clinician, who must both be willing to try to seek consensus, to share information, and to recognise each other's expertise. While the clinician has technical information, the patient knows about his or her own preferences, values, lifestyle, and so on.

However, consultation time is short, patients often find it difficult to ask the right questions, and clinicians do not necessarily know all the answers. The process therefore requires some support and traditionally, this support takes the form of patient information.

A King's Fund review of patient information material in the NHS revealed that the quality is generally poor.[1] For example, topics relevant to patients are often omitted; technical terms are used but not explained; there is incomplete coverage of treatment; and material is often inaccurate, out of date or biased. It is vital, therefore, that the quality of information to aid decision-making is improved. Some work in this area is now in progress to develop suitable materials and to evaluate their effect on, for example, the doctor–patient relationship. Preliminary results are encouraging and suggest that better informed patients are able to make sensible decisions, do not demand more and more information (as some clinicians fear), and do not increase but may even reduce clinician's workload.

But information materials alone will not solve the problems we need to address. There is a need to take a radical look at how professionals are trained. Professionals need to learn how to offer information, how to answer patients' questions, how to elicit their preferences, how to respect their right to make choices and how to share decision-making. This could achieve a shift in culture away from 'doctor knows best', still prevalent in the NHS, towards shared decision-making. The evidence suggests that this is what patients want.

References

1. Coulter A, Entwhistle V, Gilbert D. *Informing patients: an assessment of the quality of patient information materials*. London: King's Fund, 1998.

2. Coulter A. Partnerships with patients: The pros and cons of shared decision making. *Journal of Health Research and Policy* 1997; 2: 112–21.

3. Wennberg JE, Barry MJ, Fowler FJ, Mullee A. Outcome research, PORTs, and health care reform. *Annals of the New York Academy of Sciences* 1993; 703: 52–62.

Professionals, patients and information: learning issues

Summary of a presentation by Ms Sally Tweddle, Senior CRC Fellow in Cancer Information and Education, University of Birmingham.

A project involving Glasgow, Nottingham and Birmingham Universities, Great Ormond Street Hospital and (at a later stage) the King's Fund was initiated in April 1998, funded by the Enabling People Programme. The project is not only multi-centre but also multidisciplinary, involving health professionals in public health and general practice, and experts in information science and technology, education and social science. The different perspectives afforded by the variety of disciplines involved have been interesting and helpful.

The aims of the project are to:

- identify the learning needs of clinicians and desired organisational changes to fulfil the information needs of patients and to make use of well-informed patients in the professional development of clinicians
- start to develop appropriate learning materials.

Seventy-two interviews were carried out in Glasgow, Nottingham and London with a variety of health care professionals including hospital doctors, GPs, hospital nurses and health visitors. The broad range of views obtained in these interviews was then used in a Delphi exercise designed to obtain some consensus about professional learning needs.

Results showed that learning needs and the need for organisational change could be classified in eight areas:

- placing a higher priority on patient information and education
- understanding the patient's information needs and environment
- knowing about information sources and their use
- issues of the health care team
- helping patients to understand about health care and health care information

- the right information at the right time
- emotions and information
- partnership with patients.

It is interesting to note the importance seemingly attached to emotion and information.

The issues for discussion that emerged are:

- There are increasing sources of information available for patients, some high quality and some poor quality. How can the one be differentiated from the other?
- Enabling patient learning is a wider issue than can be addressed by simply developing clinician communication skills.
- There is a need to identify learning needs of clinicians, and the organisational change required, in order to enable the learning of patients, their families and carers.

The learning issues that emerged are:

- The purpose and mechanisms for providing information. There was lack of clarity among professionals about exactly why they should provide information to patients. Mechanisms for providing information appear to be various and there was lack of understanding about the importance and significance of the way information is provided.
- Ascertaining the nature/scope of patient understanding. There were few strategies revealed in the data for, for example, accessing patients' knowledge and establishing patients' understanding at the end of the consultation.
- Controlling/supporting patients' use of other sources. There is some evidence that clinicians want to control access to information.

- The reciprocal expert/novice relationship. There was only limited recognition that the relationship between professional and patient could be changed and even reversed by patient access to information.

- Language, rules and roles. These issues were least addressed in the interviews and need to be explored more fully. Patients cannot ask questions if they do not know the language in which to ask. Similarly, rules and roles within the consultation are predominantly those which enable the professional to decide what is discussed and how.

Solutions to these problems were already evident in the practice of the health professionals interviewed but these solutions were not always recognised and there is further work to be done to identify and address the learning objectives involved.

Views from primary care

Summary of a presentation by Dr Mandy Hampshire, GP and Lecturer in General Practice.

As part of the multi-centre study (*see p.10*), interviews were carried out with GPs and health visitors in Nottingham. These provide one example of the views of clinicians about how they work with well-informed parents.

(Interviews focused on parents because in Nottingham parents have been given a personal child health record since 1992 and are, by this means, better informed.)

Postal invitations were sent to all 156 health visitors and 360 GPs in the Nottingham area. Forty-six per cent of health visitors and twenty-three per cent of GPs agreed to be interviewed. A theoretical random sample was selected for interview based on the age of the respondent and the type of area in which they worked. Eleven health visitors and ten GPs were interviewed and the interviews were taped, transcribed and coded independently by two researchers. The professionals interviewed were, admittedly, a sample drawn from those who had an explicit interest in the area.

Almost all the health visitors and GPs interviewed had experience of parents presenting them with information that they, as professionals, knew little or nothing about. This included recent news from the media, and information about new services or products, alternative therapies and rare conditions. All the health visitors and GPs interviewed thought it important to admit their lack of knowledge and offer to find out more for the patient.

The information sources used by parents rarely included the Internet and did not include any other IT sources. Only one health visitor and two GPs mentioned parents having used the Internet. More usual sources of information were television, magazines, newspapers, books and leaflets, health professionals, relatives and friends, and self-help groups.

All health visitors and GPs thought they learnt from well-informed parents. They were able to identify advantages of working with well-informed parents who:

- could be a source of information
- could be more interesting/stimulating
- could remind professionals of what needs to be done
- were more likely to be compliant
- were better able to manage illness
- were more likely to be partners in care.

On the other hand, the health visitors and GPs thought there were also disadvantages to working with well-informed parents who might:

- create more stress for health professionals
- be more of a challenge (although this can also be an advantage)
- make it difficult for the health professional to keep ahead/up to date
- have unrealistic expectations
- cause health professionals to feel de-skilled
- take more time
- be more anxious as a result of health scares in the media.

The interviews also produced information relevant to training. Only half of the health visitors and GPs interviewed had read literature on the effects of educating parents. None had done any training focusing on how to deal with informed parents or new types of information delivery.

Both professional groups were asked what training they thought would help them to meet the information needs of well-informed patients:

Health visitors

Counselling skills

Updates on current issues

Interpersonal skills

Peer observation and feedback

GPs

How to access current information/keep up to date

Communication skills

Use of the Internet

How to work in multidisciplinary teams

How to identify own education needs

Similarly, health visitors and GPs were asked what organisational changes would help them to meet the information needs of well-informed patients:

Health visitors

Access to the Internet

Guidelines on how to deal with informed parents

Access to databases with up to date information

More resources to lend to parents (e.g. videos)

GPs

Summary of information currently available to patients in the press

Rapid release of information so professionals are aware as soon as patients

More time for patients (i.e. lower list size and better remuneration)

A national standard leaflet bank

It is important to note that the GPs and health visitors interviewed frequently stressed that the needs of less well-informed patients must also be met and should not be ignored. Also, the needs of well-informed patients were only one strand among a number of priorities in their learning needs.

In summary, the Nottingham work suggests that health visitors and GPs:

- are often presented by patients with information they know little or nothing about
- think it important to admit their lack of knowledge and find out relevant information
- learn from well-informed patients
- think the advantages of well-informed patients outweigh the disadvantages have not been trained to cope with well-informed patients or new types of information delivery.

Discussion

Peter Burley, Deputy Registrar, Council for Professions Supplementary to Medicine, expressed concern about the sample of GPs interviewed in Nottingham – a random sample of GPs within the twenty-three per cent who already sympathised with the project.

Mandy Hampshire accepted that this was a weakness in the methodology. She pointed out that GPs prepared to be interviewed were inevitably those who were interested in the topic and that others who were not interested or were unsympathetic were unlikely to have agreed to an interview.

B J Hutchcroft, Consultant Physician, Chest Clinic, Northern General Hospital, Sheffield, asked where the speakers felt patients wish to position themselves on the continuum which runs from, at one extreme, a lay model of disease (uninformed) and at the other extreme, a professional model (highly informed)? While this will obviously vary from patient to patient, it is critical to our understanding about what and how much patient education needs to be provided.

Angela Coulter suggested that interesting pointers are emerging from current work to evaluate the use of NHS Direct. NHS Direct is receiving increasing numbers of 'second opinion' calls – that is, calls from people who have received advice about treatment and who want to obtain more information and explore possible alternatives. This seems to suggest that people are moving towards, or want to understand more about, the medical mode of thinking about disease and illness. However, in interviews carried out by the King's Fund,[1] patients expressed a strong need to understand and make sense of illness in their own terms. It is clear that there is a culture change in progress. Numerous surveys have shown that younger people have higher expectations in relation to, for example, information, understanding and participation than older people. This is not an age effect but a cohort effect: that is, it reflects a social change which affects medical care in the same way it affects other areas of our lives.

Having said that, it is important to recognise that all patients are different, and that patients face very different situations. A patient's response in, say, a life-threatening situation may be very different to their response when, for example, they are choosing what contraception to use.

Sally Tweddle added the view that language is a significant factor, which may influence where one positions oneself on the lay–professional continuum. Lay people need to be able to understand and use the language and terminology of medical professionals, in order to enter into a more equal dialogue with health care professionals.

BJ Hutchcroft argued that, conversely, health care professionals needed to be able to avoid unnecessary medical jargon in order to communicate clearly with patients.

Reference

1. Coulter A, Entwhistle V, Gilbert D. *Informing patients: an assessment of the quality of patient information materials*. London: King's Fund, 1998.

Chair's summary

Jean Mossman, Chief Executive, CancerBACUP

Ms Mossman drew out the following themes:

- There is a need for organisational change as well as individual change. Informing patients can only become an integral part of the service if we focus on the organisation and the system as much as on individual health professionals.

- There is a lack of clarity about why we should provide information to patients and about the benefits of doing so.

- There is a need to check what patients have understood and what patients' information needs are.

- There is a large amount of emerging evidence about information provision but little awareness of this evidence among health care professionals. Knowledge management is now an important issue for the NHS and requires time and resources. As an illustration, CancerBACUP answers 45,000 enquiries per year. Two full-time librarians support the oncology nurses who answer these enquiries. This level of support is essential in order to manage the large amount of new information about cancer that is constantly becoming available.

- There is a role for the media but that role is uncontrolled, and because it is uncontrolled, it can have a major impact on health professionals' workload. Service users may acquire incorrect knowledge and unreasonable expectations as a result of inaccurate information in the media.

Jean Mossman then added a story of her own:

In January, I attended the annual general meeting of the Prostate Cancer Support Association. After presentations, the meeting split into discussion groups. The group I took part in was discussing patient involvement and shared decision-making. One participant dominated this group, returning constantly to his own experience. He had been diagnosed as having prostate cancer, referred to a radiotherapist, informed about options for treatment and advised to have radical radiotherapy. He had sought a second opinion and was referred to another radiotherapist who gave him similar information and also advised him to have radical radiotherapy. He then had the radiotherapy, after which he was told that this had not removed the cancer completely, and indeed had never been expected to do so. He then sought an opinion from a surgeon with a view to having the cancer removed surgically, only to be told that, following the radical radiotherapy, this was no longer feasible. He had not been told, at the outset, that the radiotherapy would not remove the tumour and that it would prevent him from having surgery as a second option. He was understandably distraught.

In the same group, another man had gone through a similar process. He had gone to see a radiotherapist, had been informed about his treatment options, and had been told that if he chose to have radical radiotherapy, surgery would no longer be an option. He had opted to have surgery.

So in this discussion group, there was one patient who was happy with what had happened to him, and one patient who was very unhappy.

We took these two stories to a radiotherapist, who told us that people who had had radical radiotherapy could still have surgery, and to a surgeon, who told us that surgery was not possible after radical radiotherapy.

This anecdote suggests that we should be concerned not only about how the doctor communicates information but also about what information the doctor communicates. The story highlights, too, the consequences of a poor consultation: the patient did not receive appropriate information and as a result was dissatisfied and unable to trust the professionals concerned.

Work in syndicate groups (morning session)

Following the morning's presentations, the conference broke into syndicate groups which, for this part of the day, were organised according to discipline. Each group was equipped with a list of issues, with associated learning objectives, which had emerged from the interviews with clinicians in the multi-centre study. The learning objectives were expressed in the form of quotations from these interviews.

Each group was asked to discuss and prioritise the issues, selecting the three they considered should be addressed most urgently. After discussion, the groups fed back in a plenary session.

When feeding back, groups commented on what they considered to be the unsatisfactory nature of the task. For example, many participants felt that the task was important but over-simplified. Instead of being presented with a pre-selected list of learning objectives, they would have preferred to have identified objectives for themselves. Some participants also felt that the presentation of objectives in the form of clinicians' quotes was unhelpful and gave a one-sided view of patient information issues. This view did not allow for the different perspectives of the various professionals taking part in the conference, or for the patient's voice to be considered and heard.

Syndicate group A (doctors)

First priority

Issue: Basic communication skills for all

Learning objective: 'We should try to ensure that communication skills are addressed in all curricula and that courses are attended by those who need them.'

Second priority

Issue: Judging the correct level of information required by patients and families.

Learning objective: 'Clinicians should be able to judge how much information a patient needs and in what form they need it within the consultation process.'

Third priority

Issue: Consistency of information

Learning objective: 'Clinicians and the wider clinical team need to give information to patients within a framework that takes account of national and local guidelines for patient information.'

The group commented that the statements provided for discussion did not make a satisfactory starting point. They emphasised that the patient is at the centre of these issues and underlined the importance of the consultation process. They saw the clinician as not in control but constrained by their professional role to meet a given agenda.

Syndicate group B (nurses)

First priority

Issue: Continuity of information and changes in team personnel

Learning objective: 'New members of staff should receive training in the clinical team's approach to patient information.'

The group emphasised the importance of the team as the umbrella under which the clinician practices and learns. However, in general discussion other participants commented that the nature of the clinical team varies according to the nature of the problem and therefore varies almost from patient to patient. Furthermore, the team may be spread over a wide geographical area, involving, for example, those in the community as well as hospital.

Second priority (joint)

Issue: Unlearning wrong information

Learning objective: 'Clinicians need to be sensitive in their handling of patients who have been given incorrect information.'

Second priority (joint)

Issue: The emotional needs of clinicians

Learning objective: 'Clinicians need to be supported and advised on dealing with difficult patients.'

It was felt that these two latter issues link importantly with the clinician's attitude.

Syndicate group C (information specialists)

First priority

Issue: Patient information

Learning objectives: 'Staff and students need to have opportunities to learn about the information needs of patients.'
'Clinicians should give information appropriate to the psychological and social state of the patient.'
'All medical records should include a section on what the patient has been told by whom, their understanding and concerns.'
'Clinicians need ongoing training in writing in medical records, and arrangements for patient-held records.'

The group emphasised the need to develop the patient contribution to the medical record.

Second priority

Issue: Making use of alternative support mechanisms, such as patient and parent support groups

Learning objective: 'Clinicians should know when and how to make use of alternative support mechanisms.'

Third priority

Issue: New and complementary therapies

Learning objective: 'Clinicians should decide and explain to patients – based on an assessment of the evidence – how therapies might be considered/introduced into the care programme.'

The group argued that this last issue is important because patients consider it important. Clinicians should therefore know the evidence. However, this idea prompted some general discussion about whether or not complementary therapies fall within the remit of conventional medicine, and whether appropriate techniques for assessing the effectiveness of conventional medicine are applicable to alternative therapies.

Syndicate groups D and E *(professions allied to medicine, academics and educationalists)*

As a preliminary point, the group commented critically on the top-down nature of the majority of the statements/interview quotes.

First priority

This group had difficulty prioritising one issue and instead identified a large number of learning objectives which they considered related to one overarching issue, namely:

Issue: Development of clinicians' communication and interpersonal skills and understanding of their patients' experiences and needs

Learning objectives:

'Clinicians should develop skills that will enable them to learn from patients what it is like to have a disease or to live with a condition.'

'Clinicians should know how to enable patients to obtain information relevant to their needs.'

'Clinicians need to be able to communicate the level of risk associated with the diagnosis and treatment to patients.'

'Clinicians should help patients and their families to understand how assessment of diagnosis or need for treatment may change as more information becomes available, such as tests etc.'

'Clinicians should ensure that the patient's understanding is checked over time.'

'Clinical teams need to develop consistent messages about diagnosis, treatment and care.'

'Clinicians can learn and extend their clinical knowledge from patients.'

'Clinicians should be able to judge the level of knowledge held by the family.'

'Clinicians should help patients understand how the health care team works.'

'New ways of working within health organisations could be developed which make better use of well-informed patients and their carers.'

Second priority

Issue: Multidisciplinary working

Learning objective: 'Clinical teams need to develop consistent messages about diagnosis, treatment and care.'

The group emphasised the importance of consistency in different disciplines' approach to the management of illness; consistency in messages; and consistency in acknowledging uncertainty.

Third priority

Issue: Opportunities for, and breadth of, learning

Learning objectives:
'Clinicians should develop skills that will enable them to learn from patients what it is like to have a disease or to live with a condition.'
'Clinicians can learn and extend their clinical knowledge from patients.'

The group commented on the importance of learning not only 'hard' medical facts but also 'soft' information about, for example, the experience of individual patients.

Putting the learning into action

Action on issues in practice

Summary of a presentation by Dr Fiona Moss, Associate Dean, Postgraduate Medicine, North Thames.

The question posed as the conference title – 'Does my patient know more than me?' – is an extraordinary one. The answer has to be a resounding 'Yes'. But the very fact that the question is asked is revealing about how medicine has developed. Although it is self-evident that patients know more than professionals in some important respects, some professionals presumably think that the answer to this question could be 'No'.

The consultation is, or should be, a meeting between experts.[1] And if the patient is seen as another expert, the question 'Does my patient know more than me?' does not have to be asked. The patient has greater knowledge about themselves and their predicament; the clinician may have greater knowledge about their condition.

Communication skills are often viewed (and taught) as narrow and separate. But in fact, clinical skills would be meaningless without communication skills and the role of the clinician would become merely technical. Communication skills cannot be disentangled from clinical skills and should be taught to students from the beginning of medical school. These so-called soft skills should be taught as rigorously as other skills, with the potential for students being failed if they do not reach the required standard.

Three important dimensions of quality in health care (which are therefore important in education) are:

- respect; we need to teach medical students to respect their patients
- provision of 'real' information (that is, information that the patient can use)
- choice; health care is about providing people with choices about their health and

about respecting those choices, even though this may be difficult for the clinician.

When patients are listened to, choice is given and autonomy respected, the anecdotal evidence suggests that outcomes are better.

One story from my own practice which illustrates this is about Mrs Abelson (not her real name), who came to me with anaemia. When Mrs Abelson came into hospital for transfusions, it was found that she had a tumour of the kidney. Treatment for this is to remove the kidney, after which there is a reasonable chance of recovery. I went to see Mrs Abelson and she said, 'Doctor Moss, I'd like to thank you. The doctors have been excellent, the nurses have been excellent. But I'm seventy-six, my sister died in Auschwitz, my other sister died last year in the States. I'm not sure I should have this operation.' And it turned out that she wanted more information – which I could not give her. So I arranged for her to go home, and I arranged for her to see an oncologist with a particular remit to go through the pros and cons and the evidence.

At this point in the story, it is worth commenting that I was practising at the edge of what my colleagues regarded as acceptable practice. I had, after all, sent home a patient with treatable cancer. I explained that she had gone home to make a choice about whether she wanted to have the operation or not, but my colleagues did not understand the importance of this choice. The fact is that it is difficult to practice in a way that is not regarded as out of the ordinary by most clinicians.

Mrs Abelson did decide to have the operation. My guess is that she went home, made preparations, made a will and tied up her affairs. I saw her three days after the operation, literally skipping up the ward. They had never had anyone recover so quickly and she went home the next day, having had a kidney removed at seventy-six.

It is my belief that Mrs Abelson's good recovery was linked to the fact that she was able to act in an autonomous way. She was given information and was able to make her own decision to have the operation. When patients are able to make choices in this way, there is, I believe, a higher chance of a good outcome.

In support of this unashamedly anecdotal evidence, scientific evidence about the therapeutic importance of information is provided by, for example, the work of Gustafson (1999) in the USA.[2] This suggests that those patients who are given information and support have better outcomes than those who don't; and those who use this information the most are, unexpectedly, poorer and less well educated.

What action, then, is needed? First, we need to teach at the undergraduate, postgraduate and every other level that information is an integral part of the clinical package. We also need to think of information as a therapeutic necessity. People are empowered by information, and even if they do not necessarily live longer, they feel better. Lastly, we need to understand that the consultation is about guiding choice, and that the choices then made by patients should be respected. This learning needs to be taken into our medical schools: it is not a 'soft option'.

References

1. Tuckett D *et al*. *Meetings between experts*. London: Tavistock Publications, 1985.

2. Gustafson DH. Empowering patients using computer-based health support systems. *Quality in Health Care* 1999; 8.1: 49–56.

Getting patient information needs on the learning agenda

Summary of a presentation by Dr Ray Jones, Senior Lecturer in Health Informatics, University of Glasgow.

Who will champion the cause of getting patient information on the learning agenda of health care professionals? Who will be responsible? It could be an informatics expert, a communication skills expert, or the clinical teachers. The best route may be to try to involve all three.

When and how should learning take place? Should it be after basic communication skills have been learnt? Through early patient contact? At undergraduate, postgraduate or continuing professional development level, or all of these? The answer to all these questions is 'Probably'.

However, the number of new clinicians joining the workforce is small compared to those in post. I would argue, therefore, that we should concentrate on the registrars, staff nurses and equivalent posts in professions allied to medicine because these are the professionals who will influence teaching and health services for the next twenty to thirty years.

In Glasgow, we have not so far taken any initiatives at continuing professional development level. We have, however, experimented with new learning materials at undergraduate and postgraduate levels. We have recently made radical changes to the undergraduate medical curriculum, which is now founded on problem-based learning. From the first year, the students work on their communication skills and have contact with patients. They do a considerable amount of work on computer use, and some work is done on medical records. However, until now there has been no work on patient information or the patient as learner.

A lecture plus feedback has been developed in Glasgow for third year medical and nursing degree students. Medical students receive a one-hour plenary (lecture), and nurses were given a one-hour seminar.

The plenary/lecture covered:

- reasons why patients want information
- public access to health information
- systems for patient education
- the Internet
- computer-patient interviewing
- patient-held records
- computer-based personalised patient information
- the learning needs of clinicians.

E-mail feedback was then sought from the students relating to eight learning objectives, one from each of these areas. Students were asked to rank these in order of importance and also to assess how well each objective was achieved.

The response rate was poor (fifty-three out of 240 medical students and one out of sixteen nurses). In addition, the importance rankings were done correctly by only twenty-two of these respondents. Accepting these limitations, the results of the feedback were:

Rank	Learning objective (Shortened form)	Mean confidence (out of 5)
1=	(*most*) Time management. Make clear that patients' information needs are important.	3.2
1=	Patients should know reason for referral	3.3
3=	Help patient understand risk	2.9
3=	Emotion is important to successful learning	2.9

| 5 | Should know resources available and be able to explain about quality | 2.6 |

| 6 | When and how to include family. Judge level of knowledge and roles | 2.5 |

| 7= | (*least*) How to record what patients know, and approach to learning | 2.6 |

| 7= | May lead them to learn patient's experience, new clinical knowledge | 3.4 |

These results provide some useful pointers. If a learning objective is not considered important, then it is obviously important to work on motivation. Where there is a lack of confidence, there is a need to work on skills.

The Delphi exercise carried out by colleagues at the King's Fund (*see p.10*) developed these rankings further. Two findings from the Delphi exercise are of particular interest:

- First, while the Glasgow study suggested that clinicians with poor communication skills should be 'moved' to positions in which these skills were of less importance, the Delphi exercise elicited disagreement with this idea. And yet, two out of every three respondents in the Delphi study considered there should be regular testing of communication skills. The question follows: why test communication skills if you are not prepared to act on the results?

- Second, there was uncertainty among respondents in the Delphi study about whether it was useful to employ computer systems to provide information for patients. This needs further exploration. Were respondents unsure about the evidence for using such systems? Or is this old-fashioned Ludditism?

In teaching in this area, we use the published literature. There are a number of interesting papers. For example, a group in the Netherlands developed and found successful the use of a protocol which integrated medical nursing with other information and which aimed to improve the continuity of the information received by patients.[1]

And, of course, motivation is all-important. A GP who runs communication skills courses and who participated in the Glasgow interviews commented:

> *The sad thing about it is that the ones who are good and interested are the ones who come on all the courses, and the ones who could do with coming on the courses don't see they have a need to do it, because they don't have enough insight.*

Although this comment was made about practising GPs, it is also relevant for undergraduates.

A Glasgow medical student suggested that our eight learning objectives (see above) could be summed up by the statement: 'Clinicians should use the brains they were given, and behave like decent human beings.' We have to find ways of demonstrating to this student and others that if it were this obvious and easy, patients would be more satisfied and more informed than they are.

In conclusion, if we wish to get patient information onto the learning agenda, key questions for debate are:

- What are the driving forces? They include: a good evidence base about patient information needs; patients themselves; champions such as those involved in communication skills and informatics; and getting patient information onto the audit and clinical effectiveness agenda.

- When and how should learning take place?

- How can we make organisations change in order to provide an environment that supports better patient information?

These questions should now be the focus of our discussion.

Reference

1. van Wersch A, Bonnema J, Prinsen B, Pruyn J, Wiggers T, van Geel AN. Continuity of information for breast cancer patients: the development, use and evaluation of a multidisciplinary care protocol. *Patient Education and Counselling* 1997; 30: 175–86.

Discussion

It was suggested that clinicians may have difficulty in offering choices to their patients. This is not only because they may see their role as that of a 'healer' but also because they are constrained in the choices they can offer and may be unable to meet patients' requests. Recent examples have been the prescription of Viagra, and the treatment of multiple sclerosis. It is important to recognise that choice is not simply a matter between clinician and patient but is affected by, and has to be managed within, the wider context of health policy.

Fiona Moss agreed that there is a need for the patient to understand the bigger picture. Yet the information available in the media is often flawed and this compromises the patient's understanding. It is essential that the public are given real and reliable information, not necessarily so that they can comply with the system but so that they can, if they wish, protest.

Jeanette Murphy (Senior Lecturer in Health Informatics, Centre for Health Informatics and Multiprofessional Education, Royal Free and University College Medical School) described a study carried out in 1998 by the Centre for Health Informatics and Multiprofessional Education on behalf of the UK Council of Heads of Medical Schools (CHMS).[1] The study investigated the teaching of medical informatics to undergraduate medical students and included questions about the provision of information to patients. Although the curricula of the eleven medical schools were generally found to include very little formal teaching in this area, some interesting initiatives were identified. One medical school, for example, is assessing medical students' ability to obtain informed consent from a patient, using an Objective Structured Clinical Examination (OSCE) workstation. The ability to talk to a patient and assess what information may be needed and relevant is included in clinical skills courses. Some medical school libraries have taken the lead in building collections of patient information leaflets for use in teaching.

References

1. Murphy J *et al.* How medical students learn about medical informatics: a preliminary report on the 1998 London-Scotland survey. In: Bryant J, editor. *Current Perspectives in Healthcare Computing*. Weybridge: BJCH Books, 1999: 3–16.

Work in syndicate groups (afternoon session)

Following the afternoon's presentations, the conference again broke into syndicate groups. Groupings were different to those of the morning and were multidisciplinary.

The task given to the groups was to define objectives related to:

- the learning needs of practitioners
- organisational change.

Each group was asked to address this task in relation to a specific issue:

Group A: The purpose of information exchange in the clinical consultation process.
Group B: Consistency of approach to information exchange and multidisciplinary working.
Group C: Recording information transactions.
Group D: What patients and carers know and want to know.
Group E: The availability of information sources and media for patients and carers.

Groups were asked to identify the three objectives they considered most important. After discussion, the groups fed back in a plenary session.

Group A: The purpose of information exchange in the clinical consultation process

Information exchange in the clinical consultation process should enable clinicians to:

- understand the information needs of patients
- respect the patient's values
- understand the patient's perspective.

In order to understand the purpose of information exchange, practitioners also need to understand the consultation process, what the different participants may bring to it, and the importance of the context in which the consultation takes place.

In order to bring these changes into service delivery, it is important that the organisation is involved and places value on these aspects of the consultation process. The group suggested that mentorship, reflective practice and feedback from patients were all ways in which this understanding could be developed.

Group B: Consistency of approach to information exchange and multidisciplinary working

Clinicians should:

- be able to recognise and value the information contribution of the patient
- ensure that records deliver information which is appropriate for the use of other health care professionals
- construct records with appreciation that the patient may access their own records.

The organisational changes needed would include the review and amendment of records, to make them both more consistent and more user-friendly. It is also essential that value is attached to the way patient information is expressed.

Group C: Recording information transactions

The group identified one main learning objective, namely that:

- practitioners should know how to record patients' information wants/needs in a transparent manner (possibly involving the patient) and be able to negotiate with the patient about the content.

The problem identified in relation to this objective was that there is no real language or method available for recording patients' wants and needs speedily and in a user-friendly way. Practitioners need to develop skills to enable them to record the consultation within the time available. One way of doing this might be to learn through the use of actor-patients. The role of the organisation might include the provision of IT support and the use of patient-held records.

Group D: What patients and carers know and want to know

This group identified a large number of learning objectives. These were:

- how to listen
- how to assess knowledge
- valuing patient opinion
- how to enable patients/carers to express their views
- how to build a relationship/trust/confidence with patients
- to develop understanding of the importance of patients' views
- to develop understanding of the consultation as a two-way process
- to develop self-awareness.

The organisational context needed would be one that:

- permits the admission of faults/weaknesses
- values reflective practice
- facilitates peer review
- values communication skills (for example, making time for training in communication skills as well as time for communication itself, and incorporating communication in career progression criteria)
- includes communication skills in appraisal
- involves patients at all levels of decision-making
- involves patients in training and developmental changes in the organisation
- creates posts/allocates funds to provide patient information.

The group emphasised the importance of involving the patient and hearing the patient's voice in all aspects of organisational decision-making.

Group E: The availability of information sources and media for patients and carers

Practitioners need to know that information should be broad. There are many information sources, including other people (professional or otherwise), and many different kinds and levels of information. Different sources should be recognised and patients should be helped to access them. Information should be revisited through several consultations and should be supported by guidelines for appraisal of information by both patients and professionals so that they know how to discriminate between poor and good quality information.

In order for this to happen, a clear pathway is needed for professionals to access appropriate information to share with patients. A part of this is understanding the relationships between the Centre for Health Information Quality (CHIQ), the National Electronic Library for Health (NeLH), the National Institute for Clinical Excellence (NICE), NHS Direct and other agencies.

It is also important to recognise and accommodate the socio-cultural context within which individual patients receive and use information.

Summary of the day

Professor Marshall Marinker, Visiting Professor of General Practice, The Guy's, King's College and St Thomas Hospitals Medical and Dental School, London

The day has been marked by three themes: knowledge, power and communication. Important points that have emerged under these headings are:

- First, that medical knowledge is not solid and immutable but immensely plastic. There is a significant gap between evidence-based medicine and the unique condition of the individual patient.

- Second, that health professionals may fear their ignorance and limitations and seek comfort through power and control (which some patients may even like).

- Third, that communication with patients can be manipulative, offering information, for example, which gives insight only on the professional's terms.

The consultation process has also been an important feature of the day's discussions. The traditional model of the consultation is a contract according to which the health care professional offers their own diagnosis and treatment in return for a history of the illness and access to the body of the patient. This model is far removed from the model proposed by Stacey in which the patient and doctor are seen as co-producers of health,[1] or Tuckett's description of the consultation as a 'meeting of experts'.[2] However, there is now a large amount of research evidence which can tell us about patients' experiences and we can build on this.

What mandate do we have to enter patients' lives? It is the patient's construct, and the patient's world, that count. The language of the consultation is, or should be, the language of the patient, which is a real, multi-value language, rich in ambiguity, capable of expressing the human content of the consultation. Doctors' language, or the language of science, in contrast, is a single value language which cannot therefore accommodate the patient's experienced world.

'Respect' has been a key word during the day – the mutual respect between patient and doctor. One participant in today's meeting said that through respect, we can learn from well-informed patients. But of course we can also learn from poorly informed patients and it may be as, if not more, important to do so. Is the 'well-informed patient' in fact the patient who is informed in a way of which we approve?

Another important notion has been 'honesty'. It is important to recognise that there is a cost attached to honesty, which is borne by the patient. If information is to be shared, then responsibility is also shared and the patient may or may not wish to accept this responsibility. Negotiating is therefore extremely important. In general, professionals need to think further about honesty which is fundamental in communication with patients but is often used as a gloss.

Teams and teamwork have been the subject of some debate and disagreement. Some participants have argued strongly for consistency of information among team members. While this may seem important, it is worth remembering that team members exhibit the same range of differences and the same range of cultures as patients. Absolute consistency – even if it were possible – could be highly undesirable. A degree of 'messiness' is valuable from the patient's point of view since it reveals the reality of professional uncertainty, and the differences allow space for manipulation.

Questions about education and organisational change were the starting points for the conference. Learning objectives have been identified and discussed, and there are implications here for the curricula. I would argue, however, that it is not the curricula but the teachers that need to be reformed.

The need for organisational change is very clear. The point has been forcefully made that organisations affect the way we understand and use knowledge. Traditional methods of organisation – such as the seven-minute consultation – may no longer sit comfortably with modern medicine and the needs and wants of the modern patient.

The evidence on compliance with prescribed medicines reveals the need for patient information. Some fifty per cent of patients with a chronic ongoing condition do not take their medication in optimum dosage. Similarly, the commonest cause of rejection of renal transplants appears to be failure to take the medicine. The reason for this is clear and consists in the gap between the patient's understanding and the understanding of the health professional. We need to recognise, therefore, that patient's knowledge and understanding is not a grace note in communication between patient and doctor but matters enormously.

In conclusion, the comment of the Glasgow medical student quoted earlier points the way forward:

> *All of your learning needs are essential, but you are in danger of becoming bogged down in impenetrable rhetoric. I think your eight learning objectives can be summed up by the following: clinicians should use the brains they were given, and behave like decent human beings.*

That will do for me as a summary of what we intend.

References

1. Stacey M. *Sociology of health and healing: a text book*. 2nd ed. London: Routledge, 1991.

2. Tuckett D *et al*. *Meetings between experts*. London: Tavistock Publications, 1985.

Delegate list

Juan Baeza
Research Officer, Effective Practice Programme, King's Fund

Elaine Ballard
Project Facilitator, EPP, and Senior Lecturer, University of Wolverhampton

Peter Burley
Deputy Registrar, CPSM, London

Jane Clarke
Chief Podiatrist Specialist in Diabetes, Queen's Medical Centre Nottingham

Angela Coulter
Director, Policy and Development, King's Fund

Jane Dixon
Chartered Physiotherapist and Vice Chairman, Chartered Society of Physiotherapy & Clinical Professions Information Advisory Group

Christine Doyle
Health Editor, *DailyTelegraph*

Sonia Dunn
Royal College of Speech and Language Therapists

Vikki Entwistle
Senior Research Fellow, Health Services Research Unit, University of Aberdeen

Alison Forbes
Head of Press and PR, King's Fund

Jose Garcia de Ancos

Education and Informatics Adviser, British Medical Association

Humphrey Gyde

Coordinator, Oxford and Cambridge Institute for Health Informatics

Mandy Hampshire

GP and Lecturer in General Practice, University of Nottingham

Alison Hill

Director, Effective Practice Programme, King's Fund

Alison Hughes

Senior Sister, St George's Healthcare NHS Trust, London

B J Hutchcroft

Consultant Physician, Chest Clinic, Northern General Hospital, Sheffield

Ray Jones

Senior Lecturer in Health Informatics, University of Glasgow

Gillian Jordan

Principal Lecturer, Open Learning, University of Greenwich

Glenda Kenchington

Head of Projects and Planning (Nursing), Oncology Commissioning Team, Queen Elizabeth Hospital, Birmingham

Nancy Kohner

Writer

Marshall Marinker

Visiting Professor of General Practice, The Guy's, King's College and St Thomas Hospitals Medical and Dental School, London

Alan Marr

Research Fellow, Open University

Sandra McGregor

Research Fellow, Public Health Research Unit, Glasgow

Jill Morrison

University of Glasgow

Fiona Moss

Associate Dean, Postgraduate Medicine, North Thames

Jean Mossman

Chief Executive, CancerBACUP

Beki Moult

Family Resource Manager, Great Ormond Street Hospital for Children NHS Trust

Jeannette Murphy

Senior Lecturer in Health Informatics, Centre for Health Informatics and Multiprofessional Education (CHIME), Royal Free and University College Medical School

Julia Neuberger

Chief Executive, King's Fund

Chris Pearson

Programme Manager, Clinicians Programme, Solihull Healthcare NHS Trust

David Percy

Director, Education & Training, NHSE, London

Caryl Plewes

Programme Administrator, Enabling People Programme, Solihull Healthcare NHS Trust

Helen Raison

Clinical Research Associate, Sowerby Centre for Health Informatics at Newcastle, Newcastle General Hospital

Robina Shah

The Mental Health Foundation, London

Sally Shanley

Macmillan Breast Care CNS, Newham General Hospital

Marjorie Talbot

PhD student, Nursing Informatics (Family & Child), Centre for Health Informatics, University of Wales

Sarah Thompson

Visiting Fellow, Policy and Development Directorate, King's Fund

Sally Tweddle

Senior CRC Fellow, Cancer Information and Education, University of Birmingham

J G Williams

Chairman, Clinicians Programme (EPP), School of Postgraduate Studies in Medical and Health Care, Morriston Hospital, Swansea

Rob Wilson

Research Associate, Sowerby Centre for Health Informatics, University of Newcastle